Isabel Cabrera
Adriana Polo
Natalia Valdivieso Emilia Quevedo

# VIBRATION DEVICES IN ORTHODONTICS

AF773476

Isabel Cabrera
Adriana Polo
Natalia Valdivieso Emilia Quevedo

# VIBRATION DEVICES IN ORTHODONTICS

## Biological foundations, clinical evidence and contemporary applications for the acceleration of orthodontic treatment

ScienciaScripts

**Imprint**

Any brand names and product names mentioned in this book are subject to trademark, brand or patent protection and are trademarks or registered trademarks of their respective holders. The use of brand names, product names, common names, trade names, product descriptions etc. even without a particular marking in this work is in no way to be construed to mean that such names may be regarded as unrestricted in respect of trademark and brand protection legislation and could thus be used by anyone.

Cover image: www.ingimage.com

This book is a translation from the original published under ISBN 978-620-8-82837-0.

Publisher:
Sciencia Scripts
is a trademark of
Dodo Books Indian Ocean Ltd. and OmniScriptum S.R.L publishing group

120 High Road, East Finchley, London, N2 9ED, United Kingdom
Str. Armeneasca 28/1, office 1, Chisinau MD-2012, Republic of Moldova, Europe
Managing Directors: Ieva Konstantinova, Victoria Ursu
info@omniscriptum.com

Printed at: see last page
**ISBN: 978-620-6-72178-9**

Copyright © Isabel Cabrera, Adriana Polo, Natalia Valdivieso Emilia Quevedo
Copyright © 2025 Dodo Books Indian Ocean Ltd. and OmniScriptum S.R.L publishing group

*VIBRATION DEVICES IN ORTHODONTICS*

*BIOLOGICAL FOUNDATIONS, CLINICAL EVIDENCE AND CONTEMPORARY APPLICATIONS*

*CONTEMPORARY APPLICATIONS FOR THE ACCELERATION OF ORTHODONTIC TREATMENT.*

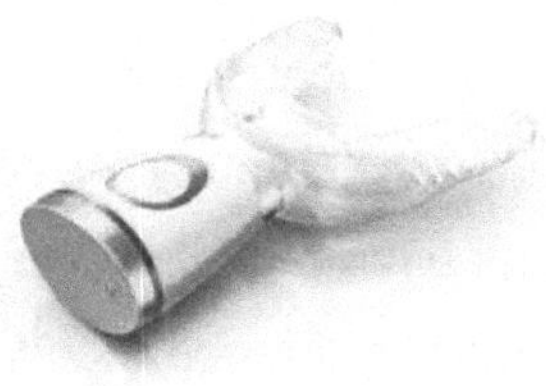

*FIGURE 1: VIBRATION DEVICES IN ORTHODONTICS HTTPS://WWW.BORDONCLINIC.COM/ACELERAR-EL-TRATAMIENTO-DE-INVISALIGN/*

# SUMMARY

Orthodontic treatments often last for months or years, resulting in patient discomfort and associated risks such as root resorption or periodontal disease. In response to this problem, various techniques have emerged to accelerate tooth movement, including the use of vibration devices. This chapter reviews the biological basis of orthodontic movement, the mechanisms of action of mechanical vibration, the available devices and the clinical evidence. Although vibratory devices offer a non-invasive alternative with some therapeutic potential, the current clinical evidence is ambivalent and does not allow a recommendation for their widespread use. The need for multicentre research, standardisation of protocols and personalised cost-benefit evaluations is emphasised.

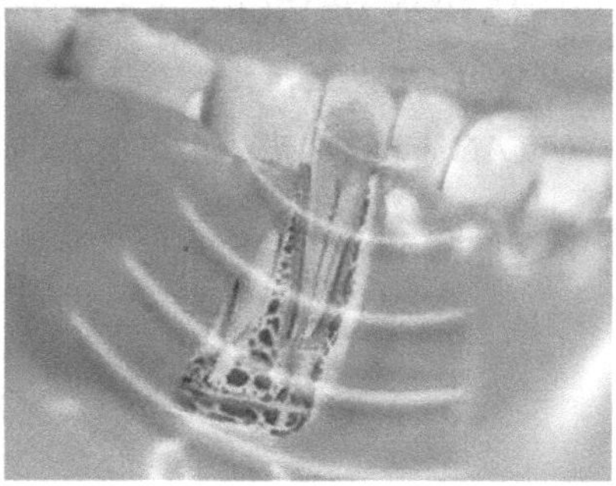

Figure 2: Vibration produced by orthodontics

https://ortodental.com.mx/tecnologia/conoce-pulsate-pro-y-acelera-tu-orthodontic-treatment/

Keywords: orthodontics, treatment acceleration, vibratory devices, bone remodelling, tooth movement.

# 1. INTRODUCTION

Orthodontic treatment generally lasts between 12 and 18 months, although this time may be longer or shorter depending on several factors. These include the complexity of the case, the type of malocclusion, the biological response of the patient, the need for other treatments beforehand and, very importantly, the level of commitment and cooperation of the patient with the orthodontist's indications (1-3).

This prolonged time is often one of the main concerns of patients, as it involves frequent visits, constant use of braces and a long wait to see the final results. However, it is also a cause for concern for practitioners, as the longer the length of treatment, the greater the risk of developing problems such as root resorption (loss of part of the tooth root), caries, gum inflammation, enamel demineralisation and other complications that can affect oral health and the success of treatment (2-4).

Concerns about the lengthy duration of orthodontic treatment have prompted the need to reduce this period with the aim of increasing the speed of tooth movement by using pulsatile forces; this approach aims to mitigate or manage the associated side effects, as well as provide greater patient safety (1,2).

There are various modalities for accelerating tooth displacement, including surgical, biological and physical methods; however, surgical approaches, although effective, are often considered invasive and, consequently, less preferred by patients (2). Biological procedures, on the other hand, involve the administration of inflammatory mediators that stimulate bone resorption, although these substances require daily systemic administration or local injections (1,2).

Vibration devices used in the orthodontic area represent a non-invasive method, characterised by their simple application and high patient acceptance (5). It has been observed that these devices allow greater movement by reducing frictional resistance to sliding, promote bone remodelling and, in addition, have the advantage of reducing pain once the patient is in the orthodontic area, They also have the advantage of reducing pain after activation of orthodontic appliances (1,6).

It is necessary to take into account that orthodontic movement is given by anabolic and catabolic effects that occur sequentially on the compression side and on the tension side, osteoblastic cells will start to produce inflammatory mediators that are related to bone resorption such as interleukins, tumour necrosis factor, forces are induced in the periodontal ligament by induction of osteoclasts and activation of RANK/RANKL (2,3).

Orthodontic tooth movement represents a complete remodelling of dentoalveolar biological tissue, involving a variety of mechanisms to achieve the desired goals (7). A fundamental theory is that of pressure-tension, which involves the application of mechanical forces capable of compressing the periodontal ligament, reducing blood flow on the compressed side (8). In areas under compression, osteoclasts themselves are activated to facilitate movement in the desired direction through bone resorption, while in regions under tension, osteoblasts are activated to promote the formation of bone trabeculae in the direction of the applied force (7-9).

Vibration devices act by stimulating the RANK/RANKL pathways and deliver cyclic forces directly to the teeth; to regulate this physiological response, orthodontic treatment combined with these devices is divided into two: high and low frequency vibration devices (2,3,6).

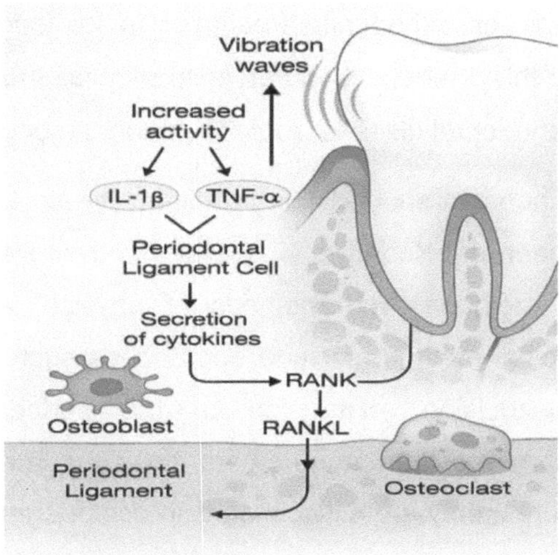


Figure 3: Orthodontic movement by anabolic and catabolic effects.

Vibration devices generate randomly varying frequencies within the range of 30-120 Hz, with an oscillating force between 0.2 N and 0.6 N, and are therefore classified into high-frequency devices, which operate at frequencies equal to or above 90 Hz, and low-frequency devices, which operate at frequencies equal to or below 45 Hz (3,10).

These devices generate vibrations or micro pulses to apply controlled cyclic forces and their indications for use are generally 20 minutes per day (11). Particularly high frequency devices induce more anabolic and catabolic alterations within the alveolar bone and the catabolic impact arises from a synergistic increase in the inflammatory response in the periodontal ligament subjected to sustained compressive forces, resulting in increased proliferation of osteoclasts facilitating tooth movement (11).

Typically, these appliances have a mouthpiece and a vibratory source, so that the vibration force reaches the teeth when the mouthpiece is bitten (12).

The disadvantage of orthodontic treatment is its long duration, and associated with this there is a great possibility of problems such as dental caries, periodontal disease, root resorption, among others (1,5).

Faced with the need to shorten this prolonged treatment time, various methods have been developed to accelerate tooth movement, including drugs, surgical methods, and methods of physical and mechanical stimulation. Surgical methods include approaches such as corticotomy, corticization, piezocision, distraction of the periodontal ligament, interceptive bone reduction, among others; however, in addition to being invasive procedures, they are associated with postoperative pain and are costly (2,5,6).

Biological procedures include the injection of exogenous inflammatory mediators and hormones that induce bone resorption; however, these substances require daily systemic administration or local injections and cause discomfort for the patient due to their recurrent applications (2,5,6).

In terms of physical and mechanical stimulation, there are several methods such as the application of direct electrical currents, laser therapies, but the most widely accepted is mechanical vibration; however, this is a controversial issue (5).

The use of vibration devices is a recent method that aims to accelerate tooth displacement during orthodontic treatment and, moreover, to reduce pain after appliance activation (2,6).

Vibration waves differentiate osteoclasts and haematopoietic cells by increasing blood flow; this is due to the fact that these waves act directly on the cell membrane and create a mechanism for inducing inflammatory mediators, which improves orthodontic tooth movement (5,6). Vibration devices are an accepted method by patients, offering advantages such as pain reduction and, most importantly, non-invasiveness (2). For this reason, it is of utmost importance to investigate vibration devices as an adjuvant factor in orthodontic treatment, regardless of the type of appliance used by the patient, with the aim of informing the scientific and general population as to whether these devices generate a significant acceleration in orthodontic movement.

## 1.1 Objectives

General Objective:

To evaluate, by review of the literature, whether the use of vibration devices contributes to a significant acceleration in orthodontic movement during treatment.

Specific Objectives:

- To determine whether high frequency devices significantly accelerate orthodontic movement.
- To evaluate the effect of low frequency devices on the acceleration of orthodontic movement.

Diagram 1: Biological cascade of tooth movement

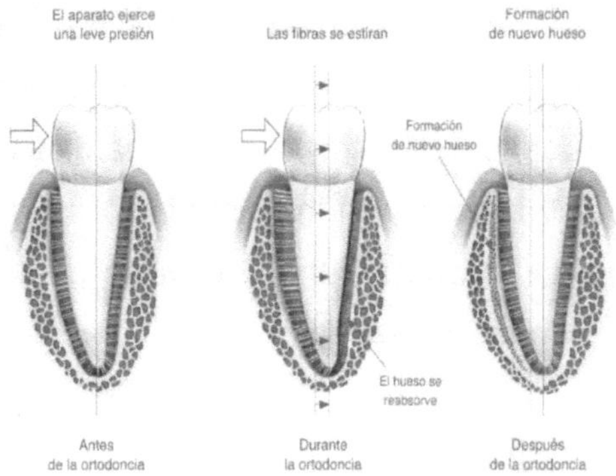


Figure 4: Biological mechanism of orthodontic movement

https://clinicaortonova.com/los-movimientos-dentales-con-ortodoncia/

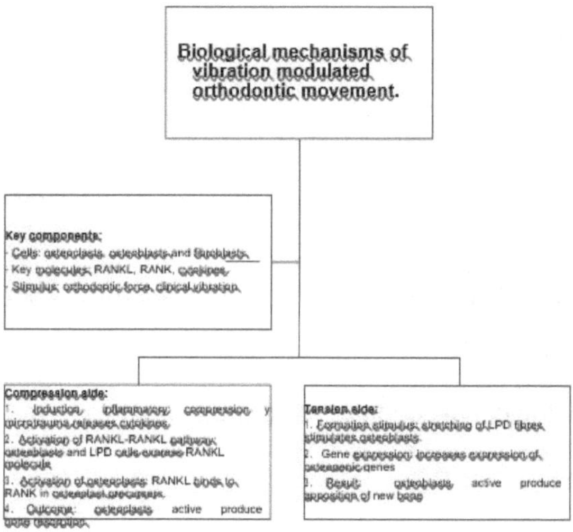


Source: Own elaboration

# 2. BIOLOGICAL FUNDAMENTALS

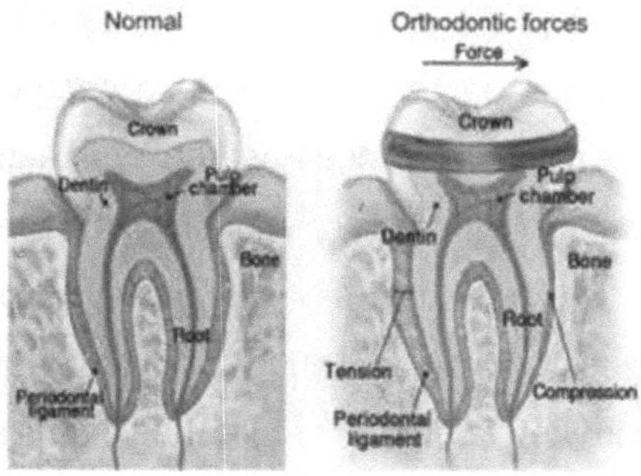


Figure 5: Biological alterations associated with orthodontics
https://www.cell.com/heliyon/fulltext/S2405-8440%2824%2908904-7

## 2.1 Orthodontic acceleration techniques

There are various techniques aimed at accelerating orthodontic movement, which fall into three main groups: surgical, biological and physical (13).Surgical techniques are the most invasive approach and are usually applied when other methods are ineffective, especially after the bone growth period is over. One of the most commonly used interventions is corticotomy, which consists of making controlled cuts in the cortical layer of the alveolar bone with the aim of inducing a temporary local osteopathy. These mechanical stimuli, such as incisions, activate the RANK/RANKL molecular pathway, which is fundamental in bone remodelling (1,13). On the other hand, micro-osteoperforations involve small transmural perforations in the bone through the mucosa. This procedure accelerates tooth movement and, being minimally invasive, reduces soft tissue damage. Moreover, it can be combined with corticotomy to enhance its effect (13).Secondly, biological techniques, also known as pharmacological therapies, aim to modulate the activity of osteoclasts and osteoblasts. Among the most commonly used is growth hormone (GH or somatotropin), which stimulates the proliferation and differentiation of osteoblasts, promoting bone remodelling. Likewise, the application of vitamin D, in its active form 1,25- dihydroxycholecalciferol, exerts an anabolic effect on bone tissue. In a complementary manner, parathyroid hormone (PTH) enhances osteoblastic activity (1,13).Finally, physical techniques are based on stimuli that increase the cellular metabolism of the tissues involved in tooth movement (3). Within this group, electromagnetic fields stand out, which modify the permeability of cell membranes and are used for procedures such as space closure, intrusion, traction of impacted teeth or palatal expansion (13). Another widely investigated method is mechanical vibration, which increases the rate of bone remodelling. Vibrations can be classified according to their frequency: low or high, each with specific effects on bone tissue (3,10,13).

## 2.2 Biological basis and mechanisms of action. Effects on alveolar bone and periodontal ligament.

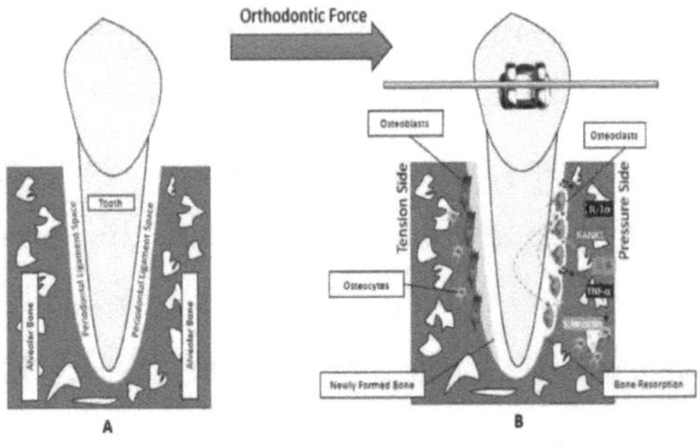


Figure 6: Model of orthodontic tooth movement.

https://www.mdpi.com/2227-9032/6/4/134

In the field of orthodontics, the application of vibration devices has emerged as an adjuvant technique to accelerate tooth movement. These devices transmit microvibrations to the dentoalveolar complex, which are picked up by the cells of the periodontal ligament and the alveolar bone. Such mechanical stimulation is essential, as these cells are directly responsible for regulating the processes of proliferation, differentiation and ultimately the tissue remodelling necessary for orthodontic displacement (14). The biological response of periodontal tissues to vibration therapy is dependent on a number of physical parameters. Firstly, the frequency and intensity of the vibratory stimulus, whether high or low, are determinant in the activation of cell signalling cascades. On the other hand, the magnitude of acceleration and the duration of stimulus application are critical factors modulating the response of the periodontal ligament and alveolar bone (14).

### 2.2.1 Alveolar Bone Level Effects

Scientific evidence shows that mechanical vibration exerts significant effects on alveolar bone, manifesting itself mainly in three areas:

- **Cell proliferation:** an increase in the population of osteoblasts, the cells responsible for the formation of new bone matrix, is observed. It is relevant to mention that the magnitude of this effect may vary depending on the vibration device used, with a more pronounced response reported with systems such as the vpro5.

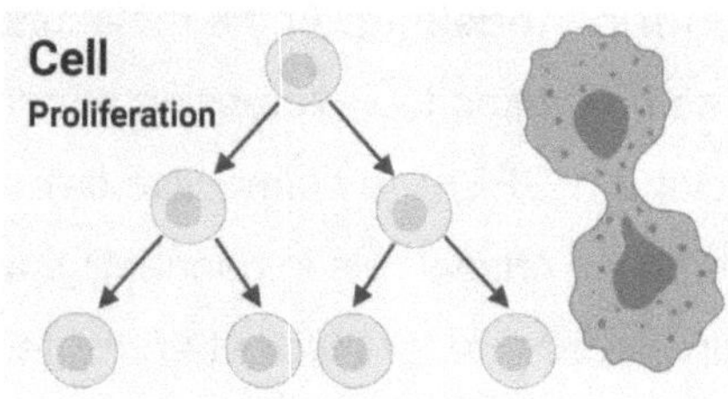


Figure 7: Cell proliferation

https://images.app.goo.gl/fZgDAChwXUfi9KUd6

- **Osteoblastic gene expression:** Vibrational stimulation induces an increase in the expression of key genes for osteogenic formation and differentiation. These include the collagen type I gene (COL1A1), the alkaline phosphatase gene (ALPL) and the transcription factor RUNX2, all key markers of osteoblastic activity (14).
- **Modulation of osteoclastic activity:** Vibration also influences the cells responsible for bone resorption, the osteoclasts. A moderate increase in osteoclastic activity has been documented, mediated by the regulation of genes such as PI3K, RANK and NFATC1, which is an essential component in the bone remodelling process that facilitates tooth movement (14).

### 2.2.2 Impact on the Periodontal Ligament

In parallel, the periodontal ligament, a key structure in mechanotransduction, actively responds to vibrational stimuli. The main effects focus on:

- **Stimulation of fibroblasts:** These cells, the most abundant in the periodontal ligament, show a clear proliferative response to vibration, contributing to adaptation and maintenance of tissue integrity during treatment.
- **Molecular activity for remodelling:** At the molecular level, vibration has been identified as promoting the expression of genes such as fibroblast growth factor 2 (FGF2) and connective tissue growth factor (CTGF). Both genes play a crucial role in connective tissue remodelling, ensuring the plasticity necessary for efficient and safe orthodontic movement (14).

In summary, although there are multiple approaches to the acceleration of orthodontic movement - including surgical and biological techniques (13) - the following approaches are available

In recent years, interest has progressively focused on less invasive physical methods such as mechanical vibration. As detailed above, the rationale for this technique is not merely mechanical, but profoundly biological, inducing a coordinated remodelling response in periodontal tissues (14). Such a response includes activation of bone formation by osteoblasts, modulation of resorption by osteoclasts and stimulation of fibroblasts in the periodontal ligament. It is therefore the understanding of these cellular and molecular mechanisms that positions vibration as a sophisticated therapeutic alternative, differentiating it from other methods by its strong biological basis and minimal invasive profile (1, 3, 10, 13, 14).

## 2.3 Proposed mechanisms:

### 2.3.1 Mechanism of Action of Vibration Induced Microtrauma.

The application of controlled mechanical vibrations induces microtrauma in the alveolar bone, a process that triggers an inflammatory response essential for tissue remodelling. This biological response is first characterised by the release of key pro-inflammatory cytokines, such as interleukin-1 beta such as interleukin-1 beta (IL-1β) and tumour necrosis factor alpha (TNF-α). As a consequence, these cytokines stimulate osteoclast activity, thereby promoting the bone resorption necessary to facilitate tooth movement (1, 2, 3). In this way, vibration therapy non-invasively simulates the biological effects of conventional orthodontic movement, with the potential advantage of accelerating the speed of treatment (1, 3).

### 2.3.2 Increased blood circulation:

The vibratory stimulus exerts a positive effect on periodontal tissue haemodynamics by improving local blood perfusion. This increased blood flow optimises the delivery of oxygen, nutrients and pro-inflammatory cells to the site of bone remodelling. As a result, this phenomenon contributes to the acceleration of cell turnover and bone matrix reorganisation (1,4).

However, the current level of evidence for this mechanism needs to be contextualised. While studies in vitro and in animal models report promising results, clinical evidence in humans attesting to its efficacy is still limited. Further research is therefore required to confirm and quantify the impact of this mechanism in orthodontic practice (3,6).

Therefore, the described mechanisms support the use of vibration as an accelerator of orthodontic treatment. The combination of a controlled inflammatory cascade (1-3) with improved tissue haemodynamics (1,4) creates a biological environment conducive to more efficient bone remodelling. However, it is crucial to recognise that clinical evidence conclusively supporting these effects in humans is still limited, a point that will be discussed in more detail below (3,6).

## 3. COMMERCIALLY AVAILABLE VIBRATION DEVICES

In the field of orthodontics, the use of vibratory devices becomes relevant as a complementary strategy to accelerate tooth movement. The two systems most commonly used in current clinical practice are the acceledent® (orthoaccel Technologies Inc., Bellaire, Texas) and the vpro5® (Propel Orthodontics, Ossining, New York). Both devices apply mechanical vibrations to the dentoalveolar complex to generate biological effects that promote bone remodelling. Although they share this principle of action, they differ in key technical characteristics such as frequency, amplitude and application time, variables that directly influence cellular response and thus therapeutic efficacy (14).

### 3.1 Acceledent®

The acceledent® device represents one of the first systems applied for orthodontic purposes. This device works by emitting low-frequency vibrations (30 Hz) with a displacement amplitude of 140 micrometres (µm). Its protocol for use establishes a daily application of 20 minutes, which, according to the evidence, reduces treatment time by 30-40 % and helps to reduce the perception of pain associated with adjustments (6,15). From a biomechanical perspective, the device achieves a total resultant acceleration of approximately 0.24 g (13,14). On a biological level, the acceledent® increases osteoblast and fibroblast proliferation, although evidence suggests that this stimulation is of moderate intensity compared to newer technologies (10,14,15).

### 3.2 Vpro5®

The vpro5® represents a technological evolution in this field, operating with high frequency vibrations (120 Hz) and a significantly smaller displacement amplitude (14 µm). Consequently, its use protocol requires only 5 minutes per day, which optimises patient comfort and adherence to treatment (14,16). This system generates a higher total acceleration of 0.41 g (13,14,16). Current scientific evidence demonstrates that vpro5® not only stimulates cell proliferation more intensely, but also induces increased gene expression associated with bone remodelling, resulting in potentially more effective acceleration of tooth movement (13,14).

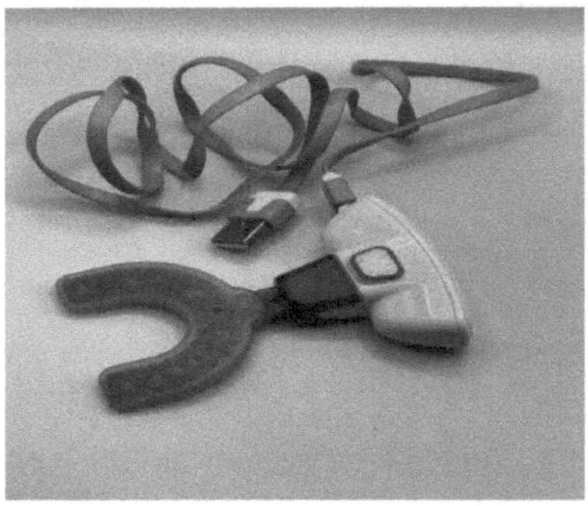

Figure 8: The vpro5® https://images.app.goo.gl/w7BWuFYbQkWAT65Z9

### 3.3 Comparative Analysis

Both acceledent® and vpro5® devices are based on the same principle of mechanotransduction to facilitate bone remodelling. However, their technical approach and their biomechanical and biological outcomes differ substantially.

First, they operate at opposite ends of the frequency and amplitude spectrum. Acceledent® uses a low-frequency, high-amplitude model, while vpro5® is based on a high frequency with minimal displacement amplitude.On the other hand, these differences result in a different biomechanical and biological impact. The vpro5® generates a significantly higher total acceleration, which, according to studies, correlates with a more robust cellular response and gene expression, suggesting a greater potential for tissue remodelling (13,14).

Finally, from a clinical perspective, their protocols for use differ markedly. The shorter daily application time of vpro5® (5 minutes vs. 20 minutes) represents a considerable advantage in terms of patient convenience and adherence. In conclusion, while both systems prove beneficial in reducing treatment time and pain, current evidence suggests that the high-frequency approach of vpro5®, combined with its greater acceleration and ease of use, may confer superior efficacy, especially in aligner protocols (13-16).

Table 1: Comparison of Technical Parameters

| Technical Parameters | Acceledent® | Vpro5® |
| --- | --- | --- |
| Frequency | 30 Hz | 120 Hz |
| Amplitude | 140 µm | 14 µm |
| Time of use | 20 minutes | 5 minutes |

Source: Own elaboration: Own elaboration

In summary, this section establishes that the two main vibratory devices in clinical practice, acceledent® and vpro5®, operate under markedly different technical principles despite sharing the same therapeutic objective. While acceledent® employs a low frequency, high amplitude model that requires prolonged daily use, the vpro5® is based on a high frequency, low amplitude approach that drastically reduces application time. This technical divergence results in a superior biomechanical impact by the vpro5®, which generates a higher acceleration and, consequently, a more intense cellular and gene stimulation. Therefore, although both systems are shown to be effective in reducing treatment time and pain, current evidence suggests potentially greater efficacy and better patient adherence with the high-frequency model of vpro5® (6, 10, 13-16).

# 4. CLINICAL EVIDENCE

The application of vibration devices as a method of accelerating orthodontic movement has been the subject of numerous clinical studies, systematic reviews and randomised clinical trials.

Several randomised clinical trials (rcts) have evaluated the effect of vibration on tooth movement velocity. Yildiz et al. (2023) reported a significant increase in canine retraction rate by low frequency vibration compared to the control group (5). Similarly, Khera et al. (2022) found greater efficiency in orthodontic movement using a customised vibratory device compared to patients who did not use it (10). Shipley et al. (2019) observed that the application of high-frequency vibration not only increased the rate of tooth movement, but also the surrounding bone density, suggesting an additional benefit on periodontal stability (13).

## 4.1 Results on tooth movement acceleration

Some clinical studies have reported positive results regarding tooth movement acceleration. Yildiz et al. observed in a controlled clinical trial that the use of vibration contributed significantly to accelerate the movement of the upper canines during the retraction phase (5). On the other hand, Khera et al. conducted a prospective study with a customised vibratory device and found a moderate increase in orthodontic movement velocity, suggesting potential benefits in well-planned treatment (10).

## 4.2 Effects on pain reduction

In addition to speeding up treatment, some studies have examined the effect of vibration on pain perception. Taha et al. conducted a pilot clinical trial in which patients who used vibration during canine retraction reported less perceived pain compared to the control group (19). This finding is complemented by the results of Toyama et al. who explored the involvement of interleukin-6 (IL-6) in the orthodontic inflammatory process and its relationship to pain. Vibration could modulate this inflammatory pathway, thus reducing discomfort during treatment (9).

### 4.3 Controversies and limitations

Despite favourable findings in some studies, controversies persist. Vega et al. and Aljabaa et al. agreed on the high variability between investigations, heterogeneity in methodological designs, small sample sizes and lack of uniformity in application frequencies and timing as key limitations that make it difficult to draw definitive conclusions (3, 6). These limitations need to be overcome by well-designed multicentre studies in order to establish clinical guidelines with greater certainty.

Table 2: Results of the level of effectiveness of the use of vibration devices in orthodontic treatment.

| Title Type of Sample Level of effectiveness study | | | |
|---|---|---|---|
| Performance comparison of vibration devices on orthodontic tooth movement tooth movement - A systematic review and meta-analysis (2). | Review Systematic Review and Meta-analysis. | 12 systematic review articles and a meta-analysis was performed on 8 of them. | There was a significant increase in the amount of tooth movement in patients using vibratory devices. |
| Effect of high-frequency vibration on orthodontic tooth movement and bone density (13). | Observation study on | 30 patients | The use of the high-frequency vibration devices during treatment with aligners significantly accelerated tooth movement movement, allowing faster completion than patients who did not undergo the use of these devices. |

| | | | |
|---|---|---|---|
| | | | the use of these devices. |
| Vibrational Force on Accelerating Orthodontic Tooth Movement: A | Review Systematic review and meta-analysis | 19 systematic review studies and were performed a meta-analysis on | 8 of 13 studies showed no significant differences in the rate of |
| Systematic Review and Meta-Analysis (14). | | The database of 4 clinical trials. | Movement dental movement with vibratory force.<br>In terms of the results<br>of the meta-analysis were inconsistent. |
| Effectiveness of using a Vibrating Device in Accelerating Orthodontic Tooth Movement: A Systematic Review and Meta-Analysis (15). | Review Systematic Review and Meta-Analysis | Seven articles were included in the systematic review and meta-analysis was performed on three of them. | 5 of the randomised clinical trials found no significant rate of significant acceleration atusing vibratory devices, only one found that it significantly accelerated movement.<br>The results of the meta-analysis no demonstrated no efficiency in the rate of acceleration of dental displacement when is used vibratory devices. |
| Comparative assessment of the rate of orthodontic tooth movement in adolescent patients undergoing treatment by first bicuspid extraction and en mass retraction, associated with low-frequency mechanical vibrations in passive self-ligating and conventional brackets: A randomized controlled trial (16. controlled trial (16). | Randomised controlled trial | 65 patients | No significant acceleration was observed after application of low frequency vibratory force. |

| | | | |
|---|---|---|---|
| Does low-frequency vibration have an effect on aligner treatment? A single-centre, randomized controlled trial (17). | Randomised controlled trial | 45 patients 3 groups: Group A: Treatment with conventional aligners | There was no significant difference in movement accuracy between group A and group C. In group B there was a better accuracy in the rotation of the |
| | | with replacement every 14 days Group B: aligners replaced every 14 days plus 20 min per day of low-frequency vibration Group B: aligners replaced every 14 days plus 20 min per day of low-frequency vibration C: aligners replaced every 7 days plus 20 minutes per day of low frequency vibration. | The upper incisors were reduced by 10%. Group B shows a better recision of the inclination of the upper canines and upper molars compared to group C. |
| Effectiveness of vibrational forces on orthodontic treatment: A randomized, controlled clinical trial (18). | Randomised, controlled clinical trial. | 20 patients | No significant difference in tooth movement rates when using vibratory devices. |
| Effects of mechanical vibrations on maxillary canine retraction and perceived pain: a pilot, single-center, randomized-controlled clinical trial (19). | Clinical trial | 21 patients | There was no significance in the rate of canine retraction when using vibrational devices. |
| Effects of vibrational devices on orthodontic tooth movement: A systematic review | Systematic review | 6 studies | One of the 6 randomised trials showed a significant acceleration in orthodontic |

| | | | |
|---|---|---|---|
| (6). | | | movement. orthodontic movement. |
| Randomized clinical trial on the effect of intermittent vibrational force application during orthodontic treatment with aligners on RANKL and OPG concentrations in crevicular fluid (20). | Randomised clinical trial | 45 patients | Intermittent vibratory force did not show significant acceleration; however, the application of vibration was associated with an increase in RANKL. |
| Effect of customized vibratory device on orthodontic tooth movement: A prospective randomized tooth movement: A prospective randomized control trial (10) | Trial prospective randomised control trial | 30 patients | No significant acceleration was found after application of low frequency vibratory forces. |
| Are Mechanical Vibrations an Effective Alternative to Accelerate Orthodontic Tooth Movement in Humans? A Systematic Review (3). | Systematic Review | 15 studies | 4 articles show significant acceleration following the use of vibratory forces, but in general vibration devices do not appear to generate a significant increase in acceleration at the orthodontic treatment. orthodontic treatment. |
| Effect of vibration on orthodontic tooth movement in a double blind prospective randomized controlled trial (21). | Prospective, randomised, controlled trial | 23 patients | Static orthodontic force supplemented with high-frequency vibratory forces for 3 min.significantly accelerated the movement at the canine retraction. |

| | | | |
|---|---|---|---|
| A different method to accelerate orthodontic tooth movement: Randomized controlled trial (5). | Randomised controlled trial | 20 patients | The application of vibratory forces in treatment with a fixed orthodontic appliance (Hycon) significantly increased the speed of tooth movement. of the the speed of tooth movement, allowing faster closure of the extraction space. extraction space. |

Source: Own elaboration

The evidence provided by the 14 articles, which include observational studies, controlled clinical trials and meta-analyses, shows varied results about the effectiveness of the use of vibratory devices on dental displacement during orthodontic treatment. devices on tooth displacement during orthodontic treatment. Five of these articles report a significant increase in the rate of acceleration of tooth displacement through the use of vibration devices (2,5,13,17,21). In contrast, the remaining nine articles report that, although vibration devices influence tooth movement, the acceleration obtained is not statistically significant (3,6,10,14-16,18-20). Specifically, of the five articles reporting a significant increase, three employ low frequency vibration devices, observing a noticeable increase in the amount of tooth movement following the application of these devices (2,5,17). The other two articles use high-frequency devices, similarly reporting that the use of these devices during orthodontic treatment significantly accelerated tooth movement (13,21). As for the remaining nine articles, four mention that a small part of their sample presented a significant acceleration of orthodontic movement after the application of vibratory forces; however, the majority of the sample did not show significance, so it was concluded that the application of vibration devices does not increase the rate of acceleration of tooth movement (3,6,14,15). On the other hand, five articles indicate that there was no significance in the acceleration of tooth mobility when using vibratory devices (10,16,18-20).

### 4.4 Final discussion of contradictory findings

The scientific evidence on the efficacy of vibration devices for accelerating orthodontic movement presents a complex picture, with promising results and, at the same time, significant controversies reflected in the literature. The analysis of the findings can be organised into three main areas. Firstly, several studies report a positive impact on the speed of treatment. Yildiz et al. (2023) observe an increased rate of canine retraction with the use of low frequency vibration (5), while Khera et al. (2022) note an increase in movement efficiency with a customised device (10). Additionally, the work of Shipley et al. (2019) not only links high-frequency vibration to faster movement, but also to an improvement in surrounding bone density, suggesting a benefit for periodontal stability (13). On the other hand, research also explores the effect of vibration on the reduction of treatment-associated pain. The trial by Taha et al. (2020) shows less pain perception in patients using vibration during canine retraction compared to the control group (19). This clinical finding finds possible biological support in the modulation of inflammatory pathways such as interleukin-6 (IL-6), a mechanism suggested by Toyama et al. (2023) (9). However, despite these favourable results, the scientific literature is not unanimous. Authors such as Vega et al. (2021) and Aljabaa et al. (2018) critically point to the considerable variability in methodological designs, limited sample sizes and lack of standardisation in vibration protocols as factors that make it difficult to draw definitive conclusions (3,6). Therefore, the scientific community agrees on the need for more rigorous multicentre studies to clinically validate the real impact of these devices in orthodontic practice.

# 5. CLINICAL APPLICATION PROTOCOLS

## 5.1 Indications and contraindications:

The clinical indications for the use of vibratory devices are mainly focused on patients requiring optimisation of the total orthodontic treatment time. Their application is especially relevant during key phases such as canine retraction or space closure. It is also recommended as adjunctive therapy in clear aligner treatment to improve predictability and efficiency of tooth movement (17, 20). On the other hand, its use has specific contraindications that must be carefully evaluated by the clinician. These include the presence of active periodontal disease, a history of severe root resorption, the existence of implants severe root resorption, the existence of recent dental implants in the area of application or the diagnosis of acute temporomandibular disorders (14, 16).

## 5.2 Recommended frequency and duration:

Commercially available orthodontic vibration devices vary in their technical characteristics and recommended protocols for use. For effective clinical application, it is critical to understand the key parameters of the device, as well as guidelines for treatment duration and consistency.

### 5.2.1 Technical parameters of the device

The two parameters that differ most between commercial systems are the vibration frequency and the daily duration of application. Firstly, the vibration frequency of most devices ranges between 30 Hz and 120 Hz. For example, acceledent® operates at a low frequency of 30 Hz, while vpro5® uses a high frequency vibration of 120 Hz. Theoretically, a higher frequency allows for a more intense stimulation of the alveolar bone and periodontal ligament (1,12,13,14).

• Secondly, the recommended daily duration is directly related to the frequency. The protocol for acceledent® suggests 20 minutes of use per day. In contrast, vpro5®, thanks to its higher frequency, requires only 5 minutes per day. This difference is based on the hypothesis that a higher frequency produces a more efficient tissue stimulation in a shorter period of time (10,13,20).

### 5.2.2 Application protocol and adherence

The effectiveness of the treatment depends not only on the parameters of the device, but also on the correct implementation of the protocol over time. Continuous use of the device is recommended throughout the active phase of orthodontic treatment, with special treatment, with special emphasis on critical stages such as canine retraction, space closure and initial alignment. In aligner therapy, its use is also indicated to optimise splint fit and predictability of movement (17,20). The importance of protocol consistency is supported by evidence from systematic reviews. Vega et al. (2021) find in their analysis that protocols with daily 20-minute sessions show better results in accelerating tooth movement than those with intermittent applications (3). Also, patient adherence is a determining factor, as those who use the devices regularly experience greater clinical efficiency (2,14).

### 5.2.3 Individualisation and clinical monitoring

However, despite the general recommendations, it is essential that the orthodontist individualise the parameters of the protocol. Consideration should be given to the specific characteristics of the patient, the type of malocclusion, the phase of treatment and the device being used. In addition, it is imperative to constantly monitor the clinical response to treatment through photographic records, cephalometric records and digital models in order to adjust the protocol as necessary to achieve the desired goals.

### 5.2.4 Combination with other orthodontic movement acceleration techniques

Vibration as a technique to accelerate orthodontic movement has been the subject of multiple studies, and its combination with other complementary strategies is currently being explored to enhance its effects. Some of the most studied combinations include micro-osteoperforations, low power lasers and minimally invasive surgical techniques. These combinations aim to generate a better alveolar bone response, optimising bone remodelling during orthodontic treatment.

### 5.2.5 Micro-osteoperforations (mops)+ vibration

Mops consist of small controlled perforations in the cortical bone that induce a localised inflammatory response, stimulating osteoclastic activity and accelerating bone resorption necessary for tooth movement. The combination of this technique with vibration devices can generate a synergistic effect by enhancing the release of cytokines such as IL-1β and TNF-α, and promoting cell recruitment in the periodontal ligament (1, 2, 3, 6). Some experimental studies even suggest that the simultaneous use of vibration maintains an active microenvironment for longer, prolonging the effects of the regional acceleration phenomenon (RAP) (13, 16).

### 5.2.6 Low power laser (LLLT)+ vibration

The use of low power lasers has been shown to improve osteoblastic activity, tissue regeneration and pain reduction during orthodontic treatment. Combining LLLT with vibration increases mechanical and biochemical stimulation of periodontal tissues, enhancing cell proliferation and bone remodelling. According to Keerthana et al. (2), some studies have reported greater and faster tooth movement in patients treated with both methods, although more methodological uniformity is required to validate these results clinically.

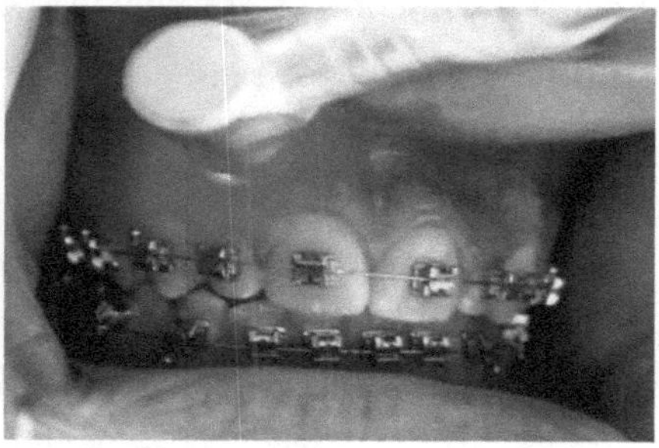

Figure 9: Low Level Laser Therapy (LLLT)
https://images.app.goo.gl/6w91GYNsqnWcHpdZA

### 5.2.7 Vibration+ minimally invasive surgical techniques

Procedures such as piezocision or minimal corticotomies, as well as mops, induce localised osteoinflammation. The addition of vibration during the weeks following surgery aims to sustain the biological activity triggered by the surgery. This combination has been described in reviews such as that of Vega et al. (3), who suggest that it may be useful for admittedly complex cases, although they stress the need for more randomised studies with prolonged follow-up.

### 5.2.8 Clinical considerations

Combinations should be carefully evaluated in each individual case, considering the periodontal status of the patient, the phase of treatment, and the type of appliance used. It is not recommended to apply multiple techniques simultaneously without clinical support, as excessive stimulation may lead to undesirable effects such as root resorption or sustained discomfort (6, 10, 16).

Table 3: Therapeutic combinations of vibration with other orthodontic acceleration techniques: effects, evidence and clinical risks.

| Combined technique | Observed effect | Clinical evidence | Potential risks |
|---|---|---|---|
| Mops+ Vibration | Synergistic acceleration of bone remodeling | Moderate | Low |
| LLLT+ Vibration | Increased cell proliferation and pain reduction | Limited | Minimal |
| Piezocision/Corticotomy+ Vibration | Prolongation of RAP, increased cell activation | Low | Moderate (surgical) |

Source: Own elaboration

## 5.3 Advantages and disadvantages

The evaluation of vibration therapy in orthodontics requires a balanced analysis of its reported benefits versus its potential limitations and risks.

### 5.3.1 Advantages of Vibration Therapy

Vibration therapy has several theoretical and clinical advantages. Firstly, from the patient's perspective, it stands out as a non-invasive and drug-free technique, which avoids systemic side effects and facilitates its application and adjustment in everyday life. Secondly, its main clinical benefit is the potential acceleration of tooth movement. This effect is attributed to several mechanisms: direct mechanical stimulation of alveolar bone (4), its potential to shorten treatment by electrical stimulation and friction reduction (1,3), and stimulation of inflammatory mediators to optimise controlled bone resorption during space closure (6).

### 5.3.2 Disadvantages and Associated Risks

However, the use of these devices also carries a number of disadvantages and risks that must be considered by the clinician and patient. Clinical and practical limitations: These include the inconsistency of results reported in the literature, the high dependence on patient cooperation to comply with the daily protocol, and the high cost of the device (1). Biological and technical risks: At the biological level, there is a potential risk of root resorption and alveolar bone fatigue if the recommended parameters of use are exceeded (4). Technically, the possibility of fatigue of the device itself is also considered, with possible variability in performance over time. Risk of bias in the evidence: Finally, a critical point is the risk of bias in the research, as some studies are sponsored by the manufacturers, which may lead to conflicts of interest affecting the published conclusions (3, 6).

## 5.4 Benefits reported by patients and orthodontists

Evaluation of vibration therapy in clinical practice involves both patient-reported outcomes and orthodontists' technical observations, presenting a nuanced picture.

### 5.4.1 Patient Perspective

Patient perception of the benefits of this therapy shows mixed results in the scientific literature. On the one hand, most studies report no statistically significant differences in pain perception, quality of alignment or overall treatment comfort (1). However, other studies indicate that patients do perceive subjective benefits, such as increased comfort compared to other acceleration methods and a feeling of reduced overall duration of orthodontic treatment (4,6).

### 5.4.2 Orthodontist's perspective

From the clinician's point of view, the evaluation focuses more on technical potential and treatment optimisation. A theoretical potential to improve the efficiency of specific movements, such as canine distalisation, is recognised, although it is stressed that success depends on the type of planned movement and the correct application of forces (1,6). Furthermore, an improvement in treatment planning is reported when the vibratory load is integrated in a precise and controlled manner with the applied orthodontic force system (4).

## 5.5 Possible adverse effects (discomfort, root resorption, device fatigue).

The application of vibration therapy is not without potential adverse effects, which should be considered and monitored by the clinician to ensure patient safety. Firstly, from the patient's perspective, the most common adverse effect is mild discomfort during use of the device (1,3,4,6). In some cases, this sensation may manifest as additional pain to the generated by the orthodontic forces (3,4,6). On a biological level, there is a potential risk of root resorption. This effect is mainly associated with an application with exaggerated parameters or in patients with a particular predisposition to this condition (1,3,4,6). Finally, on a technical level, the possibility of fatigue or malfunction of the device is considered, a risk that increases if its use is not adequately supervised by the professional (1,3,4,6).

### 5.6 Cost-benefit ratio.

The cost-benefit ratio of vibration therapy is a critical factor in clinical decision-making and presents a challenge to its widespread adoption. The high cost of commercial devices, such as acceledent® and vpro5®, contrasts with current scientific evidence. The literature reports that there is not enough conclusive evidence to routinely justify the additional cost of these appliances, given that the observed benefits are generally modest and are not consistently associated with specific phases of orthodontic treatment (1,3,4,6).

### 5.7 Future perspectives and research

To consolidate the role of vibration therapy in clinical practice, the scientific literature identifies several priority areas for further research. Firstly, studies are needed to assess the long-term effects of the daily use of these devices, as well as their real impact on the overall duration of orthodontic treatment, an aspect that has not yet been assessed. At full fully assessed (3,4,6). Secondly, a fundamental line of research is the optimisation and standardisation of protocols. This includes defining optimal parameters for vibration application (3,4,6) and standardising clinical guidelines in terms of frequency (high or low), duration of daily use and the total period of application of the stimulus(4).Finally, the specific interaction with clear aligners needs to be clarified. Studies need to be designed to differentiate the biological effect of vibration from the mechanical settling effect that these devices also produce on the splints

(3,4,6).

## 5.8 Pending areas of study (optimisation of parameters, long-term effects).

To consolidate the evidence and optimise the clinical application of vibration therapy, the scientific literature identifies several priority lines of research that remain pending.Firstly, it is essential to define the long-term effects of vibration therapy on the final outcome of treatment, including total tooth movement, future periodontal health and post-treatment stability. In parallel, further insight into the precise cellular mechanisms underlying the tissue response is required (1,4). On the other hand, one of the most important areas of study is the optimisation of the physical parameters of the stimulus. This involves rigorously determining the ideal combination of frequency, amplitude, direction and duration of vibration to maximise the therapeutic effects and minimise any potential risks (3).

## 5.9 Potential integration with other technologies (AI, telemonitoring).

The future of vibration therapy lies in its potential for integration with emerging technologies, such as artificial intelligence (AI) and telemonitoring, to create a more personalised, predictive and efficient therapeutic approach. The main avenues of integration explored in the literature are:

- Personalised monitoring and prediction: using AI algorithms to analyse real-time patient data and predict individual response to treatment, allowing for proactive adjustments (1,3,4,6).

- Automatic parameter adjustment: Develop devices capable of automatically modifying vibration parameters (frequency, duration) based on the detected biological response, thus optimising the stimulus for each patient (1,3,4,6).

• Adherence monitoring: Implement telemonitoring systems to monitor the use of the device by the patient at home, ensuring compliance with the protocol and improving the overall effectiveness of the treatment (1,3,4,6).

In summary, the clinical application of vibration therapy in orthodontics is presented as an adjunctive technique with specific indications, such as accelerating treatment and improving the efficiency of aligners (17, 20), but also with clear contraindications such as active periodontal disease (14, 16). The protocol is based on the application of vibrations with parameters that vary according to the device (e.g. 30 Hz vs. 120 Hz), and its success depends on the patient's adherence to continuous daily use (2, 3, 10, 12-14, 20). Despite its advantages - being non-invasive and drug-free (4, 6) - and its potential to be combined with other techniques such as micro-osteoperforations (1, 2, 3, 6, 13, 16), its clinical assessment is ambivalent. The evidence on its efficacy is inconsistent, with mixed perceptions from patients and orthodontists, and its high cost is often not justified by the often modest benefits (1, 3, 4, 6). In addition, it is not without risks, such as root resorption and discomfort (1, 3, 4, 6). Therefore, the future of this therapy lies in overcoming these limitations by standardising protocols, conducting long-term studies and integrating technologies such as artificial intelligence to personalise and optimise its application (1, 3, 4, 6).

# 6. CONCLUSION

## 6.1 Final reflection on the evidence reviewed

The search for methods to accelerate orthodontic movement has gained prominence in the last decade, driven by the desire to reduce treatment time and improve patient experience. Within this context, vibration devices have emerged as a non-invasive alternative, with both therapeutic and biological potential. Throughout this paper, a comprehensive analysis of the most current scientific literature on the subject has been carried out, which now allows us to establish a series of key conclusions and recommendations for clinical and research practice.

## 6.2 Summary of key findings

The findings reviewed confirm that, although vibratory devices have strong biological underpinnings, their clinical effectiveness is inconclusive. At the cellular and molecular level, multiple studies demonstrate that mechanical vibration stimulates osteoblast and fibroblast proliferation, modulates osteoclast activity and activates the RANK/RANKL pathway, which benefits bone remodelling. This physiological basis supports its use as an adjuvant technique in orthodontics.

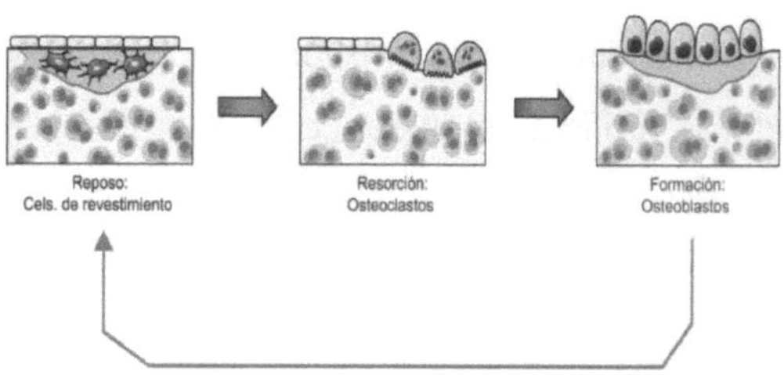


Figure 10: Osteoblast and fibroblast proliferation
https://images.app.goo.gl/2dpRv8VWZSkKoZGLA

However, when reviewing the available clinical evidence, an ambivalent picture emerges. While some randomised controlled trials report significant acceleration of tooth movement, particularly with the use of high-frequency devices such as vpro5®, other studies show no statistically significant differences. Likewise, there is notable methodological variability between studies, both in the technical parameters (frequency, amplitude, duration of use) and in the characteristics of the sample and the evaluation criteria, which conditions the generalisability of the results. Similarly, an additional benefit has been identified in terms of reducing perceived pain, possibly attributed to the modulation of inflammatory pathways such as interleukin-6. However, this effect is also inconsistent and requires further validation. In terms of clinical experience, patient adherence to the daily use protocol represents a decisive factor for treatment success. Although many patients find these devices comfortable, their consistent and disciplined use is not always achieved in real-life settings. Additionally, the high cost of the devices poses an ethical dilemma, as the clinical benefits obtained so far do not fully justify the economic investment in all cases.

### 6.3 Recommendations for clinical practice and future research

Based on the analysis, the following recommendations are made for orthodontists, researchers and students:

A) For the clinician:

- Vibration therapy should be considered as an adjunctive tool and not as part of the standard protocol. Its use should be limited to selected cases, such as treatment with aligners or canine retraction, as long as the patient demonstrates a willingness to comply with the protocol.
- An individualised assessment including periodontal history, stage of

treatment, presence of risk factors (such as previous root resorption), and patient expectations is essential.

- The decision to incorporate these devices should be accompanied by honest and ethical communication with the patient, explaining the potential benefits, the limitations of the evidence, and the cost-benefit ratio.

B) For the researcher:

- The development of multicentre clinical trials with robust methodological designs, adequate sample sizes and longitudinal follow-up is needed. Only then will it be possible to establish standardised protocols and clinical guidelines with a high level of evidence.

- Optimisation of physical parameters such as frequency, amplitude and duration remains a priority. Addressing the differential impact of these parameters will help to refine clinical application.

- It is recommended to investigate the interaction between vibration and other emerging technologies, such as digital aligner systems, telemonitoring of usage, and automatic parameter adjustment using artificial intelligence, which could transform this tool into an option customised option y more effective.

## 6.4 Final considerations

In conclusion, vibration therapy represents a captivating innovation in the field of orthodontics, combining validated biological fundamentals with a relatively simple technical application. No However, its integration into daily practice requires a critical, ethical and scientific attitude. Although the current results are encouraging in some contexts, the evidence and

limited contexts, the evidence and limited demonstration do not yet allow us to recommend its widespread use. The challenge for the coming years lies in overcoming these limitations through rigorous research, technological development and carefully monitored clinical application.

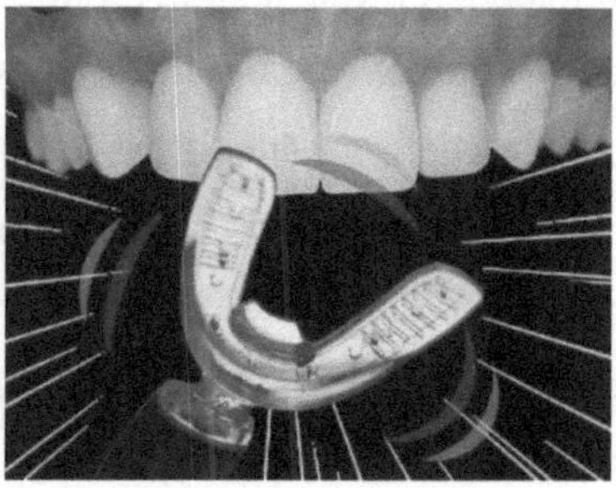

Figure 11: Orthodontic vibratory device
https://images.app.goo.gl/yEPSLg3FzEy8xpx87

### 6.4.1 Critical considerations on the use of the practice

Based on the evidence reviewed, the decision to incorporate vibration devices into daily orthodontic practice requires critical and prudent evaluation. The following are the most relevant considerations for the clinician.

### 6.4.2 Evidence of Ambivalent Efficacy

The scientific literature presents contradictory and inconclusive results. While some studies report a statistically significant acceleration of tooth movement, a considerable amount of research, including systematic reviews, finds no difference to justify its routine use. Therefore, the clinician cannot assume that the device will perform predictably in all patients.

### 6.4.3 Critical Factors: Adherence and Cost-Benefit

In addition to uncertain efficacy, there are significant practical barriers to implementation of this therapy. First, patient adherence. The success of the therapy depends critically on the patient's cooperation in adhering to a consistent daily use protocol. Since non-adherence is a common challenge in orthodontics, the practitioner must evaluate whether the patient's profile justifies the investment in a technique whose outcome depends entirely on his or her discipline. Secondly, the cost-benefit ratio. The high cost of the devices contrasts with benefits that the evidence describes as "moderate" at best and often not significant. This presents an ethical and practical dilemma, requiring full transparency with the patient about the uncertainty of outcomes before recommending further investment.

### 6.4.4 Biological Risks and Lack of Standardisation

Finally, the application of this technique is not without risks and methodological challenges. Although considered safe, there are potential risks such as root resorption if parameters are not adequately controlled. In addition, the great variability in the protocols (, duration frequency) and devices used in the studies prevents the existence of a standardised clinical guideline, leaving the responsibility for dosing in the hands of the clinician.

### 6.4.5 Clinical verdict

In short, from a critical clinical perspective, vibration therapy remains an optional adjuvant tool and not a standard of treatment. Its application should be individualised, reserved for very specific cases and highly motivated patients, always after an honest discussion about the uncertainty of its efficacy and its high cost-benefit ratio.

## BIBLIOGRAPHY


1. Leethanakul C, Phusuntornsakul P, Pravitharangul A. Vibratory stimulus and accelerated tooth movement: A critical appraisal. J World Fed Orthod. 2018;7:106-12.

2. Keerthana P, Diddige R, Chitra P. Performance comparison of vibration devices on orthodontic tooth movement - A systematic review and meta-analysis. J Oral Biol Craniofac Res. 2020;10:814-23.

3. Vega MFG, Pérez-Franco LML, Kanán AD, Méndez CDR, Sainz JES, Cervantes ER, et al. Are mechanical vibrations an effective alternative to accelerate orthodontic tooth movement in humans? A systematic review.Appl Sci (Switzerland).2021;11.

4. Jiang J, Sun J, Zeng Y, Zhang Y, Wang J, Zhou S. Determination of vibration acceleration mechanism and vibration load application duration from a non-biological perspective: Orthodontic Acceleration. Lat Am J Solids Struct. 2023;20(1).

5. Yildiz O, Yagci A, Hashimli N. A different method to accelerate orthodontic tooth movement: Randomized controlled trial. Balkan J Dent Med. 2023;27(1):51-5.

6. Aljabaa A, Almoammar K, Aldrees A, Huang G. Effects of vibrational devices on orthodontic tooth movement: A systematic review. Am J Orthod Dentofacial Orthop. 2018;154:768-79.

7. Li Y, Zhan Q, Bao M, Yi J, Li Y. Biomechanical and biological responses of periodontium in orthodontic tooth movement: up- date in a new decade.Int J Oral Sci. 2021;13.

8. Gao Y, Min Q, Li X, Liu L, Lv Y, Xu W, et al. Immune System Acts on Orthodontic Tooth Movement: Cellular and Molecular Mechanisms. Biomed Re Int.2022;2022.

9. Toyama N, Ono T, Ono T, Nakashima T. The interleukin-6 signal

regulates orthodontic tooth movement and pain. Biochem Biophys Res Commun. 2023;684.

10. Khera AK, Raghav P, Mehra V, Wadhawan A, Gupta N, Phull TS. Effect of customized vibratory device on orthodontic tooth movement: A prospective randomized control trial. J Orthod Sci. 2022;11(1):18.

11. Sangle R, Parab M, Gujare A, Dhatrak P, Deshmukh S. Effective techniques and emerging alternatives in orthodontic tooth movement: A systematic review. Med Novel Technol Devices. 2023;20.

12. Akbari A, Wang D, Chen J. Peak loads on teeth from a generic mouthpiece of a vibration device for accelerating tooth movement. Am J Orthod Dentofacial Orthop. 2022;162(2):229-37.

13. Mheissen S, Abu-Hussein M, Kaddah M. Methods of accelerating orthodontic tooth movement: A review of contemporary literature. Int J Dent Oral Health. 2018;4(4):1-8. Available from: https://www.researchgate.net/publication/326253426_Methods_of_accelerating_orthodontic_tooth_movement_A_review_of_contemporary_literature

14. Judex S, Pongkitwitoon S. Differential efficacy of 2 vibrating orthodontic devices in altering cellular response in osteoblasts, fibroblasts and osteoclasts. Dose-Response: An International Journal 2018 Jul-Sep;1-8. Doi:10.1177/1559325818792112.

15. Shipley T, Farouk K, El-Bialy T. Effect of high-frequency vibration on orthodontic tooth movement and bone density. J Orthod Sci. 2019;8(1).

16. Akbari A, Gandhi V, Chen J, Turkkahraman H, Yadav S. Vibrational Force on Accelerating Orthodontic Tooth Movement: A Systematic Review and Meta-Analysis. Eur J Dent. 2023;17(4):951-63.

17. Elmotaleb MAA, Elnamrawy MM, Sharaby F, Elbeialy AR, Eldakroury A. Effectiveness of using a vibrating device in accelerating orthodontic tooth movement: A systematic review and meta-analysis. J Int Soc Prev Community Dent. 2019;9(1):55-9.

18. Kumar V, Batra P, Sharma K, Raghavan S, Srivastava A. Comparative assessment of the rate of orthodontic tooth movement in adolescent patients undergoing treatment by first bicuspid extraction and en mass retraction, associated with low- frequency mechanical vibrations in passive self-ligating and conventional brackets: A randomized controlled trial. Int Orthod. 2020;18(4):696-705.
19. Lombardo L, Arreghini A, Huanca Ghislanzoni LT, Siciliani G. Does low-frequency vibration have an effect on aligner treatment? A single-centre, randomized controlled trial. Eur J Orthod. 2019;41(4):434-43.
20. Telatar BC, Gungor AY. Effectiveness of vibrational forces on orthodontic treatment: A randomized, controlled clinical trial. J Orofac Orthop. 2021;82(5):288-94.
21. Taha K, Conley RS, Arany P, Warunek S, Al-Jewair T. Effects of mechanical vibrations on maxillary canine retraction and perceived pain: a pilot, single-center, randomized-controlled clinical trial. Odontology. 2020;108(2):321-30.
22. Pérez Idarraga A, Yeste Ojeda F, Virto Ruiz L, Lacasa Litner M, Cacho Casado A, Martin C. Randomized clinical trial on the effect of intermittent vibrational force application during orthodontic treatment with aligners on RANKL and OPG concentrations in crevicular fluid. Bioeng Transl Med. 2023;8(3).
23. Mayama A, Seiryu M, Takano-Yamamoto T. Effect of vibration on orthodontic tooth movement in a double blind prospective randomized controlled trial.Sci Rep. 2022;12(1).
24. Sierra-Mercado M, Zavaleta-Cortijo S, Ramírez-Huayanca D. Acceleration of orthodontic movement: a review of current techniques. Rev Mex Orthod. 2020;8(2):e134-42.
25. Proffit WR, Fields HW, Sarver DM. Contemporary Orthodontics. 5th ed. Barcelona: Elsevier; 2013.
26. Srivastava K, Chugh VK. Effects of vibration on accelerating

orthodontic tooth movement in clinical and in vivo studies: A systematic review. J Indian Orthod Soc. 2024;58(1):35-44. Available from: https://www.researchgate.net/publication/382724873_Effects_of_Vibration_on_Accelerating_Orthodontic_Tooth_Movement_in_Clinical_and_In_Vivo_Studies_A_Systematic_Review/references
27. Molina-Benítez AC, Yáñez-Vico RM, Mendoza-Mendoza A, Iglesias-Linares A. Devices used in orthodontics to accelerate tooth movement: A systematic review. Dent J (Basel). 2024;12(8):243. Available from: https://www.mdpi.com/2304-6767/12/8/243
28. Fehér E, Bánkuti B, Mártonffy K, Madléna M. Vibration devices to accrate orthodontic tooth movement - a literature review. Eur J Dent. 2022;16(3):634-40. Available from: https://www.thieme-connect.com/products/ejournals/pdf/10.1055/s-0042-1758070.pdfele

**TABLE OF CONTENTS**

More Books!

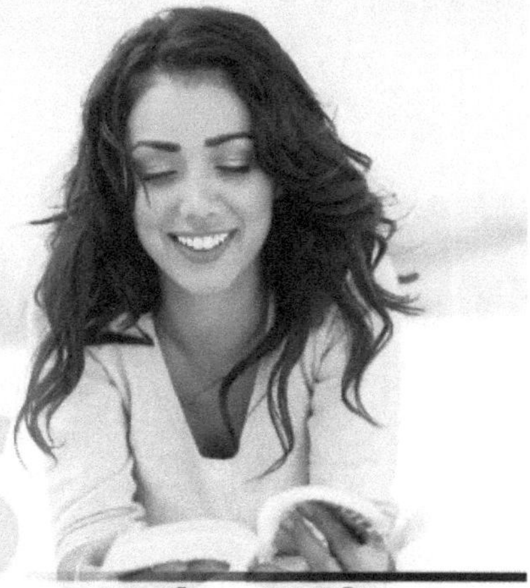

yes

I want morebooks!

Buy your books fast and straightforward online - at one of world's fastest growing online book stores! Environmentally sound due to Print-on-Demand technologies.

Buy your books online at
**www.morebooks.shop**

Kaufen Sie Ihre Bücher schnell und unkompliziert online – auf einer der am schnellsten wachsenden Buchhandelsplattformen weltweit! Dank Print-On-Demand umwelt- und ressourcenschonend produzi ert.

Bücher schneller online kaufen
**www.morebooks.shop**

info@omniscriptum.com
www.omniscriptum.com

OMNIScriptum

FSC
www.fsc.org
MIX
Papier | Fördert
gute Waldnutzung
FSC® C083411

Kolibri 360 GmbH
Ferdinand-Jühlke-Straße 7
99095 Erfurt, Deutschland
produktsicherheit@kolibri360.de

Druck:
CPI Druckdienstleistungen GmbH
im Auftrag der
Kolibri 360 GmbH
Ferdinand-Jühlke-Str. 7
99095 Erfurt